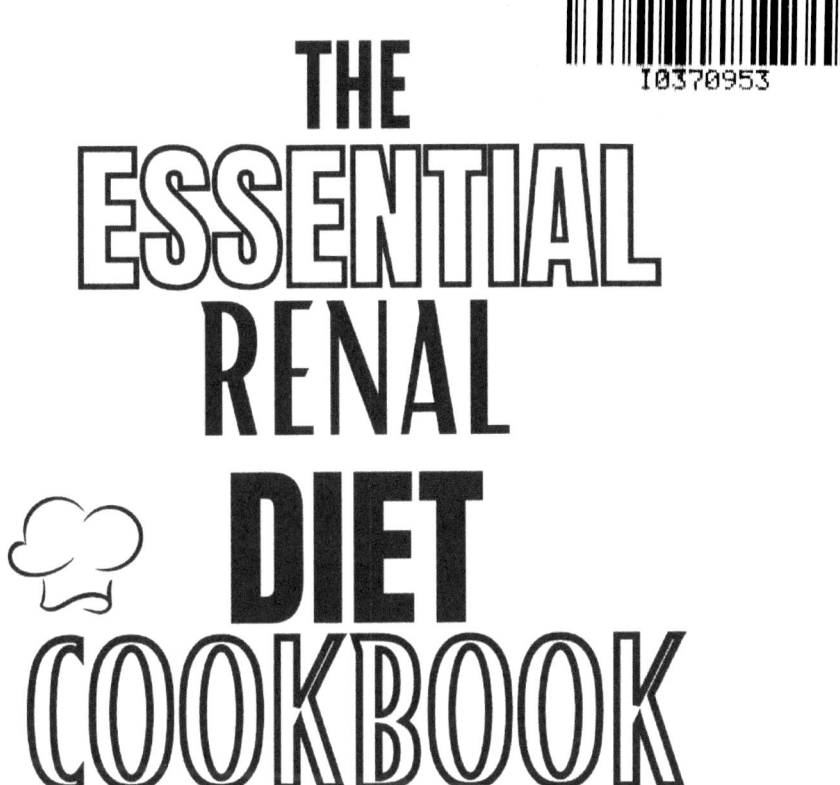

THE ESSENTIAL RENAL DIET COOKBOOK

MANAGE YOUR KIDNEY DISEASE BY FOLLOWING THESE AMAZING RECIPES

HEALTHY FOOD
PUBLISHING

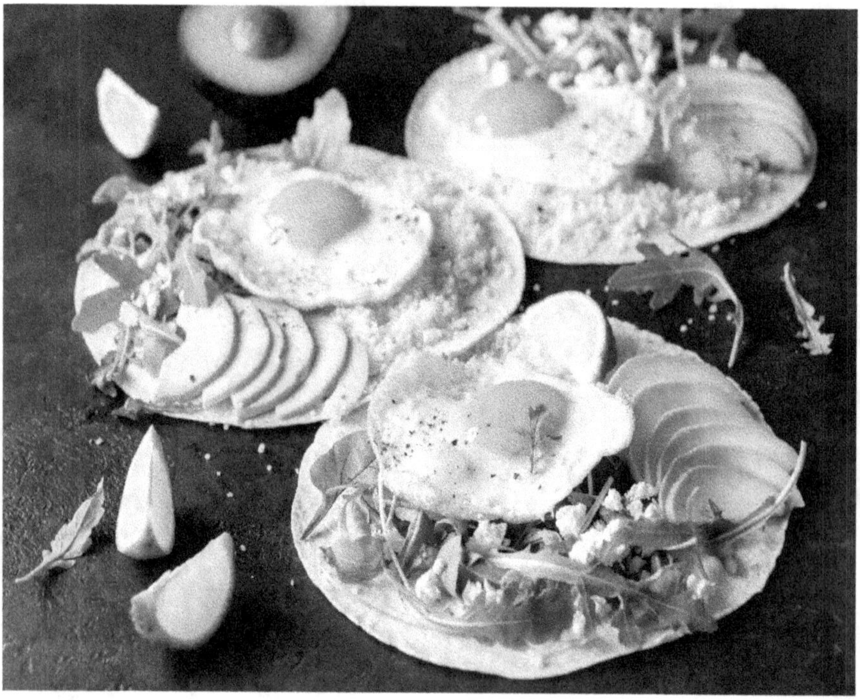

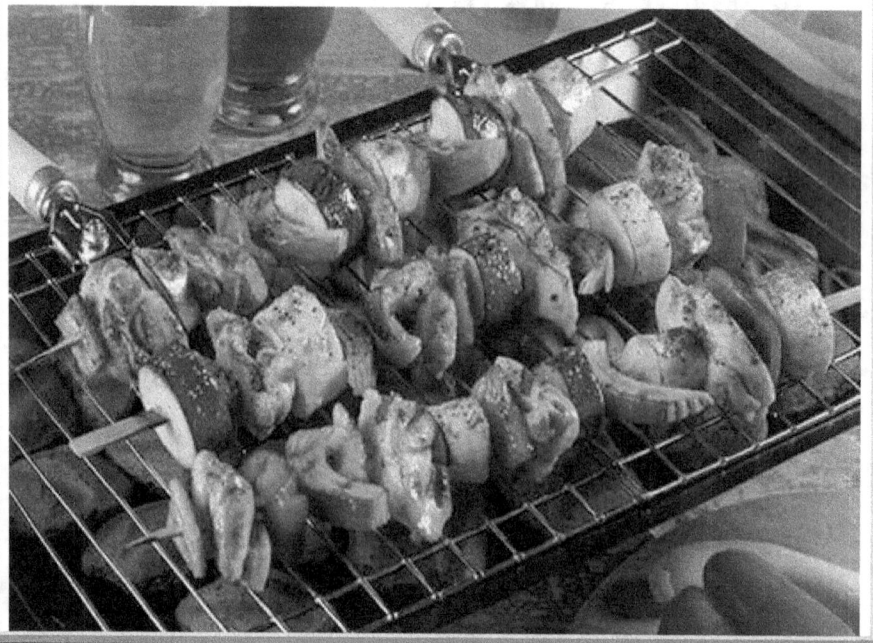

TABLE OF CONTENTS:

CHAPTER 1: BREAKFAST RECIPES 8
- COUNTRY GRAVY 9
- CREAM CHEESE AND PARMESAN BREAD SPREAD 11
- PIMENTO CHEESE WITHOUT CREAM CHEESE 13
- PASTA, BROCCOLI AND CHICKEN 15
- AVOCADO SHAKE 17
- SOUTHERN MOON PIES 19
- SIMPLE CREME BRULEE DESSERT 22
- PEACH AND RASPBERRY CRUMBLE 24

CHAPTER 2: VEGETEABLE RECIPES 27
- EASY TEMPEH SANDWICHES 28
- BRAISED CABBAGE 30
- SEASONED ROASTED ROOT VEGETABLES 32
- BREAKFAST STRATA 34
- SPRING VEGGIE BAGEL SANDWICH 37
- MACARONI SALAD 39

CHAPTER 3: POULTRY RECIPES 42
- CHICKEN VERONIQUE 43
- CHICKEN AND CHICKPEA RICE PILAF 45
- CHICKEN TERIYAKI TACOS 48
- INDIAN CHICKEN CURRY 52
- BARBECUE RIBS 55

CHAPTER 4: FISH & SEAFOOD RECIPES 58

Fish Chowder	59
Curry Fish and Rice	61
Lemon Pepper Fish Tacos	63
Oven-Baked Salmon with Herbs	65
Herb-Stuffed Baked Trout	67
Shrimp Teriyaki	69

CHAPTER 5: SALAD RECIPES 72

Bow-Tie Pasta Salad	73
Black Bean and Wild Rice Salad	75
Riced Cauliflower	77
Persimmon and Pomegranate Salad	79
Mexican Mango Salad	81
Pear Salad	83

CHAPTER 6: MEAT RECIPES 86

Rice Salad	87
Orzo and Wild Rice Salad	89
Couscous with a Kick	92
Smothered Pork Chops	94
Cheesy Pork Chops with Spicy Apples	96
Ground Beef and Chopped Cabbage	98

CHAPTER 7: SOUP & STEW RECIPES 101

Rotisserie Chicken Noodle Soup	102
Chicken Udon Noodle Soup	104
Amazing Oven-Braised Chicken Stew	106
Healthy Roasted Cauliflower Soup	109

© Copyright 2021 by Healthy Food Publishing All rights reserved.

The following Book is reproduced below with the goal of providing information that is as accurate and reliable as possible. Regardless, purchasing this Book can be seen as consent to the fact that both the publisher and the author of this book are in no way experts on the topics discussed within and that any recommendations or suggestions that are made herein are for entertainment purposes only. Professionals should be consulted as needed prior to undertaking any of the action endorsed herein.

This declaration is deemed fair and valid by both the American Bar Association and the Committee of Publishers Association and is legally binding throughout the United States. Furthermore, the transmission, duplication, or reproduction of any of the following work including specific information will be considered an illegal act irrespective of if it is done electronically or in print. This extends to creating a secondary or tertiary copy of the work or a recorded copy and is only allowed with the express written consent from the Publisher. All additional right reserved.

The information in the following pages is broadly considered a truthful and accurate account of facts and as such, any inattention, use, or misuse of the information in question by the reader will render any resulting actions solely under their purview. There are no scenarios in which the publisher or the original author of this work can be in any fashion deemed liable for any hardship or damages that may befall them after undertaking information described herein.

Additionally, the information in the following pages is intended only for informational purposes and should thus be thought of as universal. As befitting its nature, it is presented without assurance regarding its prolonged validity or interim quality. Trademarks that are mentioned are done without written consent and can in no way be considered an endorsement from the trademark holder.

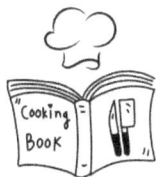

CHAPTER 1: BREAKFAST RECIPES

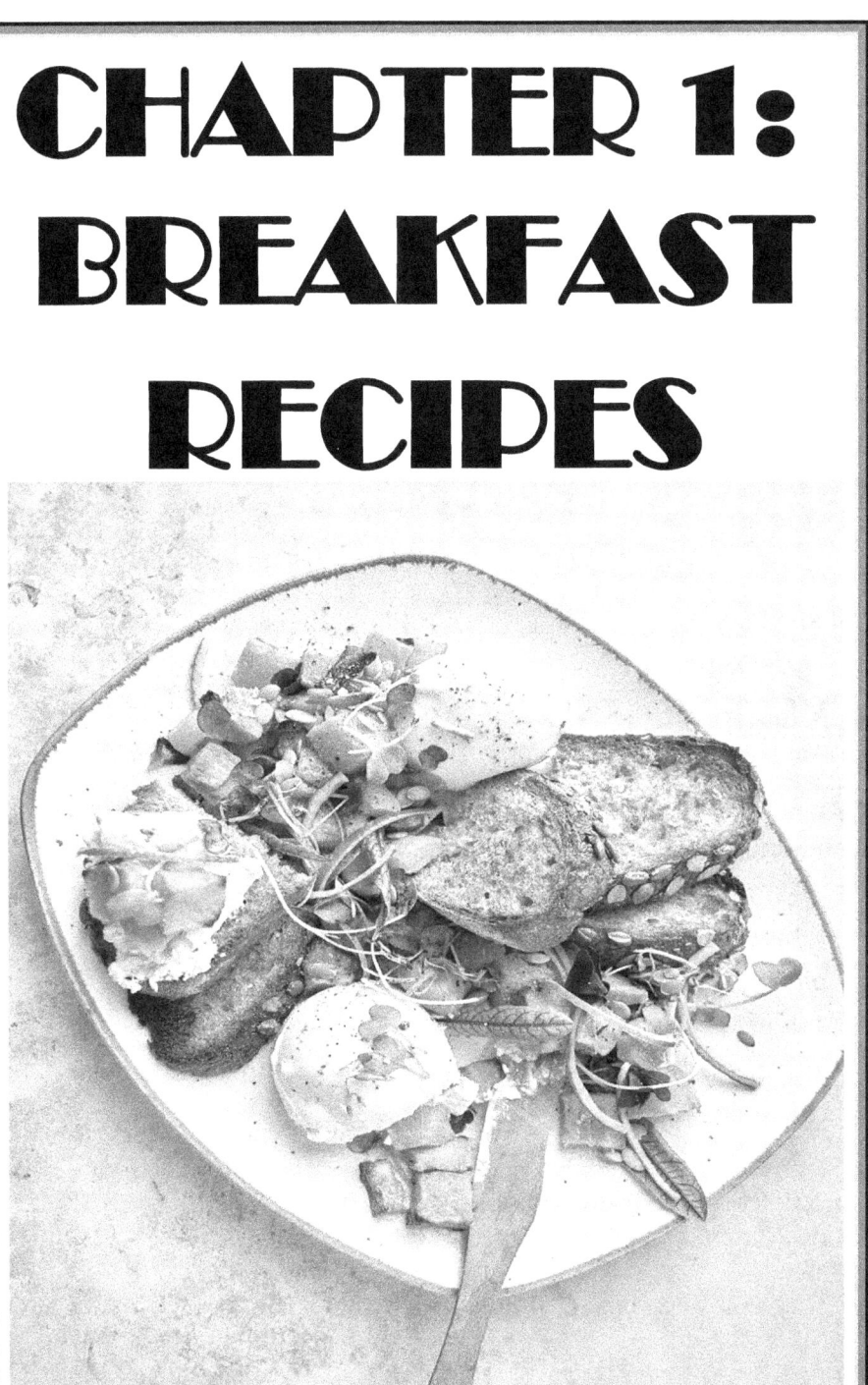

COUNTRY GRAVY

Prep:
15 mins
Cook:
35 mins
Total:
50 mins
Servings:
4
Yield:
4 servings

INGREDIENTS:

1 pinch cayenne pepper, or to taste
salt and freshly ground black pepper to taste
2 ½ cups cold milk
1 tablespoon chopped green onion
1 pinch cayenne pepper for garnish
2 tablespoons butter
8 ounces breakfast sausage links, casings removed and meat broken up
4 strips bacon, sliced crosswise
½ cup chopped green onions (light parts only)
⅓ cup packed all-purpose flour

DIRECTIONS:

1

Melt butter in a large skillet or saucepan over medium heat; cook sausage and bacon in the hot butter, stirring to break the sausage up into small pieces, until sausage is browned and bacon is almost crisp, about 10 minutes. Mix 1/2 cup green onion into sausage mixture and saute until onions are soft, about 3 more minutes.

2

Stir flour into meat mixture, 1 to 2 tablespoons at a time, until thoroughly combined and mixture is pasty. Cook, stirring often, 2 to 3 minutes to remove raw taste of flour.

3

Whisk milk into meat mixture, about 1 cup at a time, until combined. Continue to whisk until gravy begins to thicken, about 5 minutes. Turn heat to medium-high, bring gravy to a simmer, and season with a pinch of cayenne pepper, salt, and black pepper. Reduce heat to medium-low.

4

Continue to simmer gravy until flavors have blended and gravy is thick, 10 to 15 minutes, stirring occasionally. Sprinkle with 1 tablespoon green onion and a pinch of cayenne pepper for garnish.

NUTRITION FACTS:

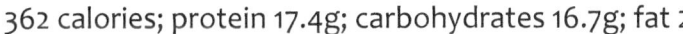

362 calories; protein 17.4g; carbohydrates 16.7g; fat 24.8g;

CREAM CHEESE AND PARMESAN BREAD SPREAD

Prep:
10 mins
Total:
10 mins
Servings:
6
Yield:
3 /4 cup

INGREDIENTS:

¼ cup Parmesan cheese
4 cloves garlic, pressed
1 ½ teaspoons Italian seasoning
½ cup softened butter
½ cup cream cheese, softened

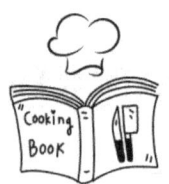

DIRECTIONS:

1
Mix the butter, cream cheese, Parmesan cheese, garlic, and Italian seasoning in a bowl until evenly blended.

NUTRITION FACTS:

222 calories; protein 3.1g; carbohydrates 1.6g; fat 23.1g;

PIMENTO CHEESE WITHOUT CREAM CHEESE

Prep:
15 mins
Total:
15 mins
Servings:
24
Yield:
3 cups

INGREDIENTS:

1 teaspoon freshly ground black pepper
½ teaspoon kosher salt
¼ teaspoon cayenne pepper
1 dash hot pepper sauce
2 cups shredded aged sharp Cheddar cheese, at room temperature
½ cup jarred pimento peppers, drained and finely chopped
¼ cup chopped green onions
½ cup mayonnaise

DIRECTIONS:

1
Combine Cheddar cheese, pimento peppers, and green onions in a medium bowl.

2
Combine mayonnaise, black pepper, salt, cayenne pepper, and hot sauce in another bowl.

3
Stir mayonnaise mixture gently into the cheese mixture using a rubber spatula until thoroughly combined.

NUTRITION FACTS:

72 calories; protein 2.5g; carbohydrates 0.6g; fat 6.8g; cholesterol 11.6mg;

PASTA, BROCCOLI AND CHICKEN

Servings:
6
Yield:
6 servings

INGREDIENTS:

1 cup chopped tomatoes
¾ cup grated Parmesan cheese
1 pound boneless chicken breast halves, cooked and chopped
salt to taste
12 ounces rigatoni pasta
½ pound fresh broccoli florets
¼ cup olive oil
1 tablespoon minced garlic
2 tablespoons pesto
ground black pepper to taste

DIRECTIONS:

1

In a large pot with boiling salted water cook rigatoni pasta until al dente. Drain.

2

Meanwhile, blanch broccoli florets in a medium size saucepan, remove with slotted spoon. In same pan saute the minced garlic and pesto sauce in the olive oil for 2 minutes. Add the chopped tomatoes and set aside.

3

In a large bowl toss cooked pasta with blanched broccoli, cooked chicken, and garlic/tomato mixture. Add grated Parmesan cheese, salt, and ground black pepper and mix well. Serve warm.

NUTRITION FACTS:

509 calories; protein 34.4g; carbohydrates 45.7g; fat 21.3g; cholesterol 67.2mg;

AVOCADO SHAKE

Prep:
10 mins
Total:
10 mins
Servings:
2
Yield:
2 shakes

INGREDIENTS:

1 ripe avocado, peeled and chopped
6 teaspoons white sugar, or to taste
1 pinch salt (Optional)
4 pods cardamom pods
2 cups cold milk

DIRECTIONS:

1

Pop cardamom pods open and crush or grind seeds into a powder.

2

Combine cardamom, milk, avocado, sugar, and salt in a food processor. Blend until smooth. Divide between 2 glasses.

NUTRITION FACTS:

332 calories; protein 10.1g; carbohydrates 32.6g; fat 19.5g; cholesterol 19.5mg;

SOUTHERN MOON PIES

Prep:
30 mins
Cook:
8 mins
Total:
38 mins
Servings:
24
Yield:
2 dozen pies

INGREDIENTS:

1 ½ teaspoons baking soda
½ teaspoon baking powder
½ cup butter, softened
1 cup confectioners' sugar
½ teaspoon vanilla extract
1 cup marshmallow creme
½ cup butter, softened
1 cup white sugar
1 egg
1 cup evaporated milk
1 teaspoon vanilla extract
2 cups all-purpose flour
½ teaspoon salt
½ cup unsweetened cocoa powder

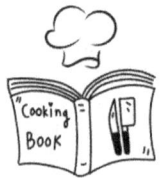

DIRECTIONS:

1

Preheat oven to 400 degrees F (200 degrees C). Lightly grease a cookie sheet.

2

To Make Cookie Crusts: In a large mixing bowl, cream together 1/2 cup butter or margarine and white sugar. Add egg, evaporated milk, and vanilla. Mix well. In a separate bowl, mix together flour, salt, cocoa powder, baking soda, and baking powder. Add flour mixture slowly to sugar mixture while stirring. Mix just until all ingredients are combined.

3

Drop the dough onto greased cookie sheet by rounded tablespoonfuls. Leave at least 3 inches in between each one; dough will spread as it bakes.

4

Bake in preheated oven for 6 to 8 minutes, until firm when pressed with finger. Allow to cool at least one hour before filling.

5

To Make Marshmallow Filling: In a medium mixing bowl, blend together 1/2 cup butter or margarine, confectioners' sugar, flavored extract, and marshmallow creme. Mix until smooth. Assemble pies by spreading 1 to 2 tablespoonfuls of filling on flat side of a cookie crust, then covering filling with flat side of another cookie crust.

NUTRITION FACTS:

193 calories; protein 2.5g; carbohydrates 26.7g; fat 9g; cholesterol 31.1mg;

SIMPLE CREME BRULEE DESSERT

Prep:
15 mins
Cook:
50 mins
Additional:
2 hrs 10 mins
Total:
3 hrs 15 mins

INGREDIENTS:

3 tablespoons white sugar
1 cup heavy cream
3 egg yolks
¼ teaspoon vanilla extract
2 tablespoons white sugar, divided

DIRECTIONS:

1

Preheat oven to 350 degrees F (175 degrees C).

2

Whisk 3 tablespoons sugar and cream in a microwave-safe bowl until well combined; heat the mixture in microwave until warm, 1 to 2 minutes, and whisk again to dissolve sugar. Whisk in egg yolks and vanilla extract until smooth.

3

Pour cream mixture into 2 ramekins. Set ramekins into a roasting pan and pour in enough hot water to reach halfway up the sides of the ramekins.

4

Bake in the preheated oven until creme desserts are set but still slightly jiggly when shaken, about 50 minutes. Remove ramekins from hot water and chill in refrigerator until cold, at least 2 hours.

5

Sprinkle 1 tablespoon of sugar evenly over the top of each dessert. Use a kitchen torch to lightly toast and melt the sugar topping until brown and bubbly, about 30 seconds. Let the sugar topping cool before serving. To serve, use a spoon to crack the crisp sugar open to reveal the creamy dessert underneath.

NUTRITION FACTS:

612 calories; protein 6.4g; carbohydrates 35.5g;

PEACH AND RASPBERRY CRUMBLE

Prep:
20 mins
Cook:
35 mins
Total:
55 mins
Servings:
10
Yield:
10 servings

INGREDIENTS:

3 fresh peaches, pitted and sliced into equal crescents
1 pint fresh raspberries
¾ cup white sugar, divided
1 tablespoon ground cinnamon, divided
1 lemon, juiced
2 cups rolled oats
1 ¼ cups all-purpose flour
½ cup unsalted butter, cubed
¼ cup brown sugar
1 teaspoon salt

DIRECTIONS:

1

Preheat the oven to 400 degrees F (200 degrees C).

2

Combine peaches, raspberries, 1/2 cup white sugar, 1/2 tablespoon cinnamon, and lemon juice in a bowl.

3

Combine oats, flour, butter, remaining 1/4 cup white sugar, brown sugar, and salt in a bowl; mix crumble topping thoroughly until smooth and not lumpy.

4

Pour fruit mixture into a large ceramic baking dish, spreading evenly. Top evenly with oat crumble mixture.

5

Bake in the preheated oven until golden brown, about 35 minutes.

NUTRITION FACTS:

305 calories; protein 4.3g; carbohydrates 50.5g; fat 10.6g; cholesterol 24.4mg

CHAPTER 2: VEGETEABLE RECIPES

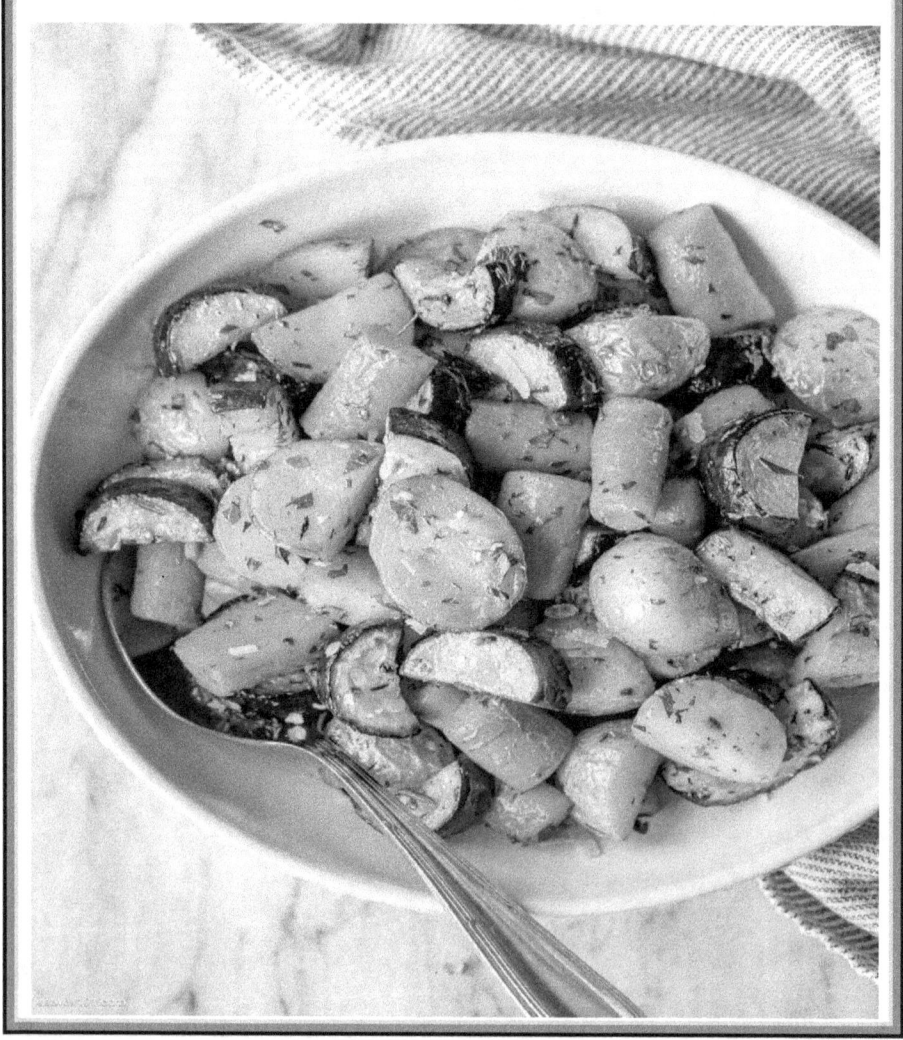

EASY TEMPEH SANDWICHES

Prep:
10 mins
Cook:
20 mins
Total:
30 mins
Servings:
4
Yield:
4 sandwiches

INGREDIENTS:

1 small onion, thinly sliced
1 medium green bell pepper, thinly sliced
1 jalapeno pepper, sliced
2 pita breads, cut in half
soy mayonnaise
4 thin slices Swiss cheese
1 tablespoon sesame oil
1 (8 ounce) package tempeh, sliced into thin strips
2 tablespoons liquid amino acid supplement
1 tablespoon sesame oil

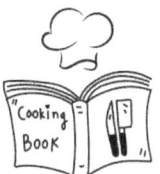

DIRECTIONS:

1

Heat the oil in a large skillet over medium heat. Add the tempeh slices and cook 3 to 4 minutes, or until they start to brown. Pour in half of the liquid aminos and cook for 1 minute. Flip the tempeh slices and cook until toasted, 3 to 4 more minutes. Pour in the remaining liquid aminos and cook for 1 minute. Remove the tempeh, and set it aside.

2

In the same skillet, heat the remaining oil over medium heat. Cook the onion, green pepper, and jalapeno until the vegetables have softened, 4 to 5 minutes.

3

Spread each pita half with 1 teaspoon soy mayonnaise. Stuff each pita with several slices of tempeh, peppers and onions, and a piece of Swiss cheese. Toast the sandwiches in a toaster oven for 2 minutes or until the cheese has melted.

NUTRITION FACTS:

392 calories; protein 21.7g; carbohydrates 24.4g; fat 24.8g;

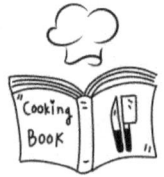

BRAISED CABBAGE

Prep:
10 mins
Cook:
25 mins
Total:
35 mins
Servings:
6
Yield:
3 cups

INGREDIENTS:

1 tablespoon white vinegar
1 tablespoon white sugar
2 teaspoons caraway seeds
1 teaspoon salt
2 tablespoons butter, or more to taste
½ head cabbage, cored and cut into 1/4-inch slices
½ onion, cut into 1/4-inch slices
1 cup water

DIRECTIONS:

1

Melt butter in a large skillet over medium heat. Cook and stir cabbage and onion until onions are translucent, about 5 minutes. Pour in water; add vinegar, sugar, caraway seeds, and salt. Reduce heat to low and cook, stirring occasionally, until cabbage is tender, 20 to 25 minutes.

NUTRITION FACTS:

77 calories; protein 1.6g; carbohydrates 9.9g; fat 4.1g; cholesterol 10.2mg;

SEASONED ROASTED ROOT VEGETABLES

Prep:
30 mins
Cook:
45 mins
Total:
1 hr 15 mins
Servings:
10
Yield:
10 servings

INGREDIENTS:

1 parsnip, peeled and sliced
3 carrots, cut into large chunks
2 tablespoons olive oil, or as needed
1 teaspoon ground thyme
1 teaspoon dried rosemary
1 pinch salt
olive oil cooking spray
1 butternut squash - peeled, seeded, and cut into 1-inch pieces
1 large sweet potato, peeled and cut into 1-inch cubes
1 (10 ounce) package frozen Brussels sprouts, thawed and halved
1 onion, halved and thickly sliced
ground black pepper to taste

DIRECTIONS:

1

Preheat oven to 400 degrees F (200 degrees C). Spray a baking sheet with cooking spray.

2

Combine butternut squash, sweet potato, Brussels sprouts, onion, parsnip, and carrots in a large bowl. Drizzle with olive oil and toss to coat. Add thyme, rosemary, salt, and black pepper; toss again. Transfer coated vegetables to the prepared baking sheet.

3

Roast vegetables in the preheated oven for 25 minutes; stir and continue roasting until vegetables are slightly brown and tender, about 20 more minutes.

NUTRITION FACTS:

149 calories; protein 3.4g; carbohydrates 29.9g; fat 3.1g; sodium 47.1mg.

BREAKFAST STRATA

Prep:
20 mins
Cook:
1 hr 15 mins
Additional:
2 hrs
Total:
3 hrs 35 mins

INGREDIENTS:

1 pound sausage, casings removed
2 cups sliced fresh mushrooms
8 eggs, beaten
10 cups cubed, day-old bread
3 cups whole milk
2 cups shredded Cheddar cheese
1 ½ cups cubed Black Forest ham
1 (10 ounce) package frozen chopped spinach, thawed and drained
2 tablespoons all-purpose flour
2 tablespoons mustard powder
1 teaspoon salt
2 teaspoons butter, melted
2 teaspoons dried basil

DIRECTIONS:

1

Generously grease a 9x13-inch casserole dish.

2

Heat a skillet over medium heat; cook and stir sausage until crumbly and completely browned, about 10 minutes. Transfer cooked sausage to the prepared casserole dish.

3

Cook and stir mushrooms in the same skillet over medium heat until liquid has been released and mushrooms are lightly browned, 5 to 10 minutes; drain.

4

Mix mushrooms, eggs, bread, milk, Cheddar cheese, ham, spinach, flour, mustard powder, salt, butter, and basil together in a large bowl; pour over sausage. Cover casserole dish and refrigerate, 2 hours to overnight.

5

Preheat oven to 350 degrees F (175 degrees C).

6

Bake in the preheated oven until a knife inserted into the center of the strata comes out clean, 60 to 70 minutes.

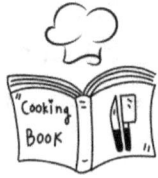

NUTRITION FACTS:

600 calories; protein 34.2g; carbohydrates 32g; fat 37.2g; cholesterol 255.6mg

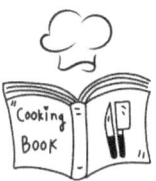

SPRING VEGGIE BAGEL SANDWICH

Prep:
15 mins
Total:
15 mins
Servings:
1
Yield:
1 sandwich

INGREDIENTS:

salt and ground black pepper to taste
1 bagel, sliced in half
3 radishes, thinly sliced
¼ cup arugula
3 slices tomato
¼ cup cream cheese
¼ teaspoon fresh lime juice
¼ teaspoon balsamic vinaigrette

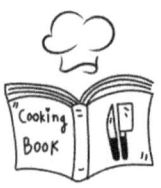

DIRECTIONS:

1

Mix the cream cheese, lime juice, balsamic vinaigrette, salt, and pepper in a bowl. Spread the mixture evenly over one of the bagel halves. Arrange the radish slices, arugula, and tomato on top of the cream cheese. Sandwich with the remaining bagel half.

NUTRITION FACTS:

381 calories; protein 11.3g; carbohydrates 36g; fat 21.7g; cholesterol 63.8mg;

MACARONI SALAD

Prep:
20 mins
Cook:
15 mins
Additional:
4 hrs
Total:
4 hrs 35 mins
Servings:
8
Yield:
8 servings

INGREDIENTS:

½ cup finely chopped green bell pepper
¼ cup finely chopped carrot
1 hard-boiled egg, chopped
2 cups elbow macaroni
¼ cup sweet relish
½ cup onion, finely chopped

Dressing:

¼ cup creamy salad dressing (such as Miracle Whip®)
2 tablespoons white sugar
1 teaspoon dried dill weed
¼ teaspoon salt
¼ cup reduced-fat sour cream
2 tablespoons low-fat milk
¼ teaspoon ground black pepper

DIRECTIONS:

1

Bring a large pot of lightly salted water to a boil. Cook elbow macaroni in the boiling water, stirring occasionally, until tender yet firm to the bite, about 8 minutes. Drain well; rinse with cold water and drain again.

2

Reserve 2 tablespoons relish juice; place the rest in a large bowl with onion, bell pepper, carrot, and egg.

3

Whisk creamy salad dressing into reserved relish juice. Mix in sour cream, milk, sugar, dill, salt, and pepper. Fold gently into the macaroni mixture. Refrigerate to let flavors blend, 4 to 24 hours.

NUTRITION FACTS:

172 calories; protein 4.9g; carbohydrates 28.9g; fat 4.1g; cholesterol 32.3mg;

CHAPTER 3: POULTRY RECIPES

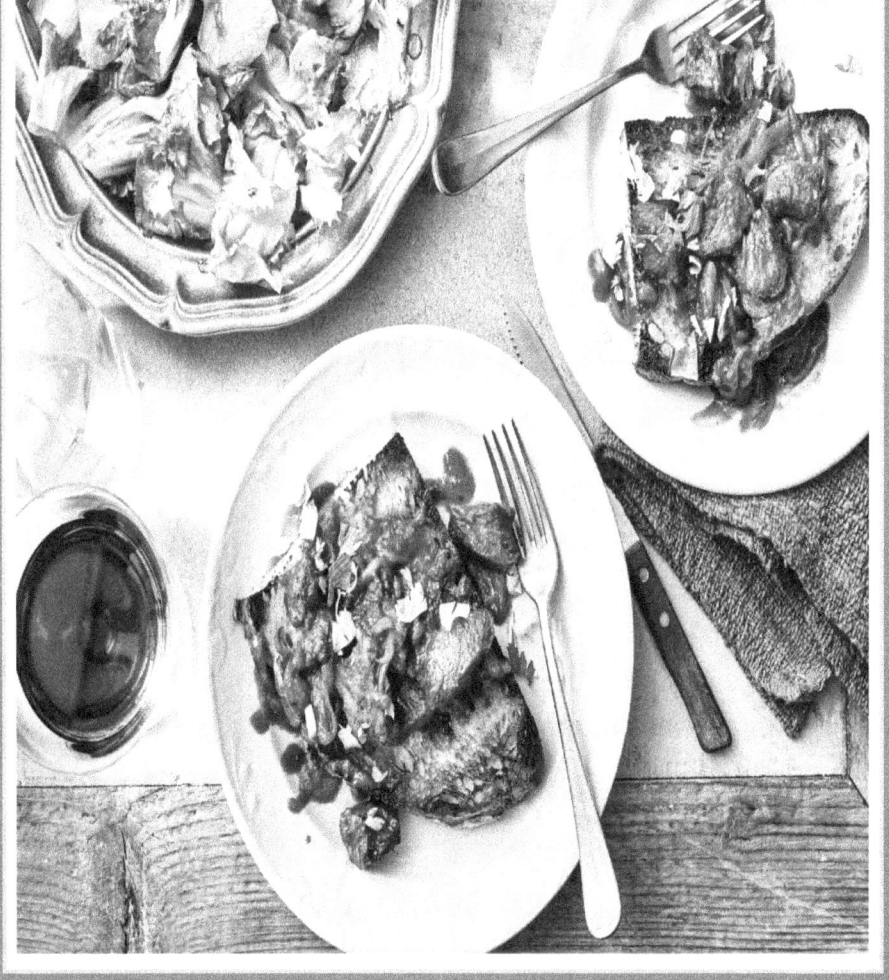

CHICKEN VERONIQUE

Prep:
20 mins
Cook:
55 mins
Total:
1 hr 15 mins
Servings:
6
Yield:
6 servings

INGREDIENTS:

1 tablespoon olive oil
1 tablespoon butter, melted
¼ cup all-purpose flour
½ teaspoon salt
2 ½ pounds chicken, cut into pieces
½ cup orange marmalade
1 cup chicken stock
1 tablespoon cornstarch
3 tablespoons lemon juice
½ cup green seedless grapes
lemon, sliced
Italian parsley, chopped

DIRECTIONS:

1

Preheat oven to 375 degrees F (190 degrees C). Pour olive oil and butter into a 9x13-inch baking dish. With a spatula, spread oil and butter to cover the bottom of the baking dish.

2

Place the flour, salt, and chicken pieces into a large resealable plastic bag, and shake to coat lightly. Arrange chicken pieces skin-side down in a single layer in the baking dish.

3

Bake in preheated oven for 20 minutes. Turn chicken pieces and bake 10 minutes. Brush chicken with 1/2 marmalade, and bake until the chicken is golden brown and fork tender, about 10 to 15 minutes. Remove chicken to a serving platter, and keep warm.

4

Reserve 2 tablespoons of drippings to a saucepan, and place over medium-high heat. Stir in chicken stock. In a small bowl, mix together cornstarch and lemon juice; stir into stock mixture. Bring to a boil, and cook until sauce thickens, 3 to 4 minutes. Stir in remaining marmalade. Stir in grapes, and cook until heated through. Serve sauce over chicken, and garnish with lemon slices and parsley.

NUTRITION FACTS:

550 calories; protein 36.3g; carbohydrates 28g; fat 32.9g;

CHICKEN AND CHICKPEA RICE PILAF

Prep:
20 mins
Cook:
1 hr 9 mins
Total:
1 hr 29 mins
Servings:
6
Yield:
1 skillet

INGREDIENTS:

6 chicken drumsticks
2 teaspoons salt, divided
2 teaspoons ground black pepper, divided
2 teaspoons ground cayenne pepper, divided
1 teaspoon dried thyme
2 cups chicken broth
1 tablespoon butter
1 tablespoon vegetable oil
1 onion, diced
1 (15 ounce) can chickpeas, drained
1 cup long-grain brown rice

DIRECTIONS:

1
Preheat the oven to 425 degrees F (220 degrees C).

2
Melt butter with oil in a large saucepan over low heat. Add onion; cook and stir until translucent, 7 to 10 minutes. Add chickpeas and cook until heated through, 3 to 5 minutes. Add rice; cook and stir until translucent and coated in oil, 4 to 5 minutes. Remove from heat.

3
Season drumsticks with 1 teaspoon salt, 1 teaspoon black pepper, and 1 teaspoon cayenne pepper.

4
Heat a large cast iron skillet over medium-high heat. Cook drumsticks until skin is golden brown and crispy on all sides, about 10 minutes. Transfer to a plate.

5
Pour chicken broth into a deep saucepan and bring to a boil. Season with remaining salt, black pepper, and cayenne pepper; add thyme. Reduce heat to a simmer.

6
Transfer chickpea-rice mixture to an oven-proof cast iron skillet. Pour in the chicken broth and mix. Place drumsticks on top and cover skillet tightly with aluminum foil.

7

Bake in the preheated oven until rice is tender, 30 to 40 minutes. Remove aluminum foil, raise oven temperature to 450 degrees F (230 degrees C); continue baking until rice is crispy on top, 10 to 15 minutes more.

NUTRITION FACTS:

343 calories; protein 24.9g; carbohydrates 37.4g; fat 10g; cholesterol 69mg;

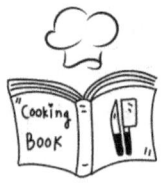

CHICKEN TERIYAKI TACOS

Prep:
25 mins
Cook:
23 mins
Additional:
25 mins
Total:
1 hr 13 mins
Servings:
6
Yield:
6 servings

INGREDIENTS:

Japanese Cucumber Salad:

3 Japanese cucumbers, very thinly sliced
1 tablespoon kosher salt
¼ cup rice vinegar
1 tablespoon soy sauce
2 teaspoons white sugar
1 teaspoon sesame oil
1 tablespoon toasted sesame seeds

Teriyaki Sauce:

3 tablespoons soy sauce
2 tablespoons mirin
2 tablespoons sake
2 tablespoons white sugar

Chicken:

1 tablespoon vegetable oil
6 bone-in, skin-on chicken thighs
Toppings:
6 (6 inch) corn tortillas
1 (8 ounce) container sour cream
3 tablespoons sriracha sauce
3 scallions, sliced into thin strips
1 tablespoon black sesame seeds (Optional)

Toppings:

6 (6 inch) corn tortillas
1 (8 ounce) container sour cream
3 tablespoons sriracha sauce
3 scallions, sliced into thin strips
1 tablespoon black sesame seeds (Optional)

DIRECTIONS:

1

Place cucumber slices in a colander in the sink. Sprinkle salt on top and toss to coat. Allow to sit for 20 minutes. Rinse cucumber slices very well with cold water; drain.

2

Mix rice vinegar, 1 tablespoon soy sauce, 2 teaspoons sugar, and sesame oil together in a bowl. Add cucumber slices and sesame seeds. Toss gently and transfer to the refrigerator.

3

Whisk 3 tablespoons soy sauce, mirin, sake, and 2 tablespoons sugar in a small bowl to make teriyaki sauce.

4

Heat oil in a large skillet over medium-high heat. Prick chicken skin all over with a fork; place skin-side down in the hot oil. Cook until the skin is golden brown, about 12 minutes. Flip and continue cooking until second side is browned, about 7 minutes.

5

Reduce heat to medium; pour teriyaki sauce over chicken. Cook until sauce thickens, about 2 minutes. Remove from heat. Cover and let rest for 5 minutes. Slice chicken into strips and place in a bowl; add teriyaki sauce from the skillet and toss to coat.

6
Toast corn tortillas in a large, dry skillet over medium-high heat until crisp and slightly blackened around the edges, 1 to 2 minutes per side. Wrap in a dish towel to keep warm.

7
Mix sour cream and sriracha sauce together in a small bowl.

8
Divide teriyaki chicken among tortillas. Drizzle sour cream-sriracha mixture over chicken. Top with cucumber salad, scallions, and black sesame seeds.

NUTRITION FACTS:

422 calories; protein 23.2g; carbohydrates 23.4g; fat 25.1g; cholesterol 87.7mg;

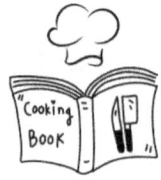

INDIAN CHICKEN CURRY

Prep:
20 mins
Cook:
40 mins
Total:
1 hr
Servings:
6
Yield:
6 servings

INGREDIENTS:

2 pounds skinless, boneless chicken breast halves
2 teaspoons salt
½ cup cooking oil
1 ½ cups chopped onion
1 tablespoon minced garlic
1 tablespoon water
1 (15 ounce) can crushed tomatoes
1 cup plain yogurt
1 tablespoon chopped fresh cilantro
1 teaspoon salt
½ cup water
1 teaspoon garam masala
1 tablespoon chopped fresh cilantro
1 tablespoon fresh lemon juice

1 ½ teaspoons minced fresh ginger root
1 tablespoon curry powder
1 teaspoon ground cumin
1 teaspoon ground turmeric
1 teaspoon ground coriander
1 teaspoon cayenne pepper

DIRECTIONS:

1

Sprinkle the chicken breasts with 2 teaspoons salt.

2

Heat the oil in a large skillet over high heat; partially cook the chicken in the hot oil in batches until completely browned. Transfer the browned chicken breasts to a plate and set aside.

3

Reduce the heat under the skillet to medium-high; add the onion, garlic, and ginger to the oil remaining in the skillet and cook and stir until the onion turns translucent, about 8 minutes. Stir the curry powder, cumin, turmeric, coriander, cayenne, and 1 tablespoon of water into the onion mixture; allow to heat together for about 1 minute while stirring. Mix the tomatoes, yogurt, 1 tablespoon chopped cilantro, and 1 teaspoon salt into the mixture. Return the chicken breast to the skillet along with any juices on the plate. Pour 1/2 cup water into the mixture; bring to a boil, turning the chicken to coat with the sauce. Sprinkle the garam masala and 1 tablespoon cilantro over the chicken.

4
Cover the skillet and simmer until the chicken breasts are no longer pink in the center and the juices run clear, about 20 minutes. An instant-read thermometer inserted into the center should read at least 165 degrees F (74 degrees C). Sprinkle with lemon juice to serve.

NUTRITION FACTS:

427 calories; protein 38.1g; carbohydrates 14.7g; fat 24.3g; cholesterol 94.7mg;

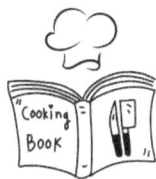

BARBECUE RIBS

Prep:
15 mins
Cook:
2 hrs
Additional:
1 hr
Total:
3 hrs 15 mins
Servings:
8
Yield:
8 servings

INGREDIENTS:

4 pounds pork spareribs
1 cup brown sugar
¼ cup ketchup
¼ cup soy sauce
¼ cup Worcestershire sauce
¼ cup rum
½ cup chile sauce
2 cloves garlic, crushed
1 teaspoon dry mustard
1 dash ground black pepper

DIRECTIONS:

1

Preheat oven to 350 degrees F (175 degrees C). Cut spareribs into serving size portions, wrap in double thickness of foil, and bake for 1 1/2 hours. Unwrap, and drain drippings. (I usually freeze the drippings to use later in soups.) Place ribs in a large roasting pan.

2

In a bowl, mix together brown sugar, ketchup, soy sauce, Worcestershire sauce, rum, chile sauce, garlic, mustard, and pepper. Coat ribs with sauce and marinate at room temperature for 1 hour, or refrigerate overnight.

3

Preheat grill for medium heat. Position grate four inches above heat source.

4

Brush grill grate with oil. Place ribs on grill, and cook for 30 minutes, basting with marinade.

NUTRITION FACTS:

504 calories; protein 29.9g; carbohydrates 23.1g; fat 30.2g; cholesterol 119.9mg;

CHAPTER 4: FISH & SEAFOOD RECIPES

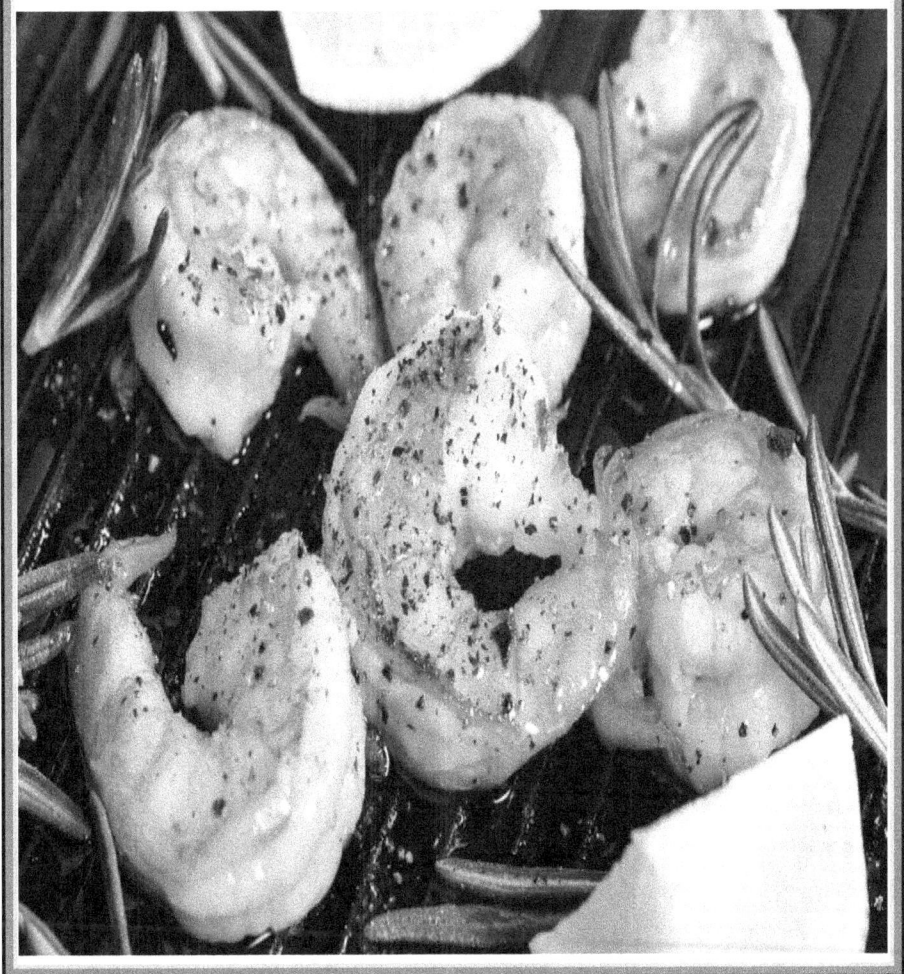

FISH CHOWDER

Prep:
30 mins
Cook:
30 mins
Total:
1 hr
Servings:
8
Yield:
8 servings

INGREDIENTS:

2 tablespoons butter
1 cup clam juice
½ cup all-purpose flour
⅛ teaspoon Old Bay Seasoning TM, or to taste
salt to taste
ground black pepper to taste
2 (12 fluid ounce) cans evaporated milk
¼ cup cooked crumbled bacon
2 cups chopped onion
4 fresh mushrooms, sliced
1 stalk celery, chopped
4 cups chicken stock
4 cups diced potatoes
2 pounds cod, diced into 1/2 inch cubes

DIRECTIONS:

1

In a large stockpot, melt 2 tablespoons butter over medium heat. Saute onions, mushrooms and celery in butter until tender.

2

Add chicken stock and potatoes; simmer for 10 minutes.

3

Add fish, and simmer another 10 minutes.

4

Mix together clam juice and flour until smooth; stir into soup and simmer for 1 minute more. Season to taste with Old Bay seasoning, salt, and pepper. Remove from heat, and stir in evaporated milk. Top each bowl with crumbled bacon, if desired.

NUTRITION FACTS:

386 calories; protein 31.9g; carbohydrates 33.8g; fat 13.6g; cholesterol 83.5mg;

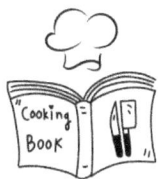

CURRY FISH AND RICE

Prep:
10 mins
Cook:
25 mins
Total:
35 mins
Servings:
4
Yield:
4 servings

INGREDIENTS:

¾ teaspoon salt
¾ cup white rice
2 frozen white fish fillets, unthawed
2 tablespoons sliced almonds
1 cup frozen peas, thawed
2 cups water
¼ cup diced onion
2 tablespoons butter
1 ½ teaspoons curry powder

DIRECTIONS:

1

Heat water, onion, butter, curry powder, and salt in a large skillet over medium heat until butter is melted, about 2 minutes. Stir rice into onion mixture and arrange frozen white fish over rice. Sprinkle with almonds.

2

Reduce heat to medium-low, cover, and simmer until the rice is tender and the liquid has been absorbed, about 20 minutes. Fish should be heated through, and the flesh should be opaque and flake easily. Mix in peas and fluff rice with a fork before serving.

NUTRITION FACTS:

344 calories; protein 21.6g; carbohydrates 34.9g; fat 12.7g; cholesterol 66.3mg;

LEMON PEPPER FISH TACOS

Prep:
20 mins
Total:
20 mins
Servings:
8
Yield:
8 tacos

INGREDIENTS:

8 hard corn taco shells, warmed
¼ tablespoon Pico de gallo
¼ tablespoon Guacamole
¼ teaspoon Sour cream
1 square Lemon Pepper Saute Starter
½ pound tilapia fillets
3 cups coleslaw mix
½ cup cilantro leaves

DIRECTIONS:

1

Melt lemon pepper square in 10-inch nonstick skillet over medium-low heat just until bubbles begin to form.

2

Add fish.

3

Saute 7-10 minutes or until golden brown on both sides and flaky. Remove from skillet.

4

Stir coleslaw and cilantro into skillet until coated and heated through.

5

Break fish into bite-sized pieces. Fill each taco shell with coleslaw mixture, fish and additional toppings.

NUTRITION FACTS:

146 calories; protein 7.4g; carbohydrates 14.5g; fat 6.5g; cholesterol 16.9mg; sodium 154mg.

OVEN-BAKED SALMON WITH HERBS

Prep:
15 mins
Cook:
15 mins
Additional:
30 mins
Total:
1 hr
Servings:
6
Yield:
6 servings

INGREDIENTS:

2 cloves garlic, finely minced, or more to taste
1 teaspoon ground coriander
salt and ground black pepper to taste
1 (2.5 pound) boneless salmon fillet
1 cup chopped fresh dill
3 tablespoons olive oil
1 lemon, juiced
1 tablespoon honey

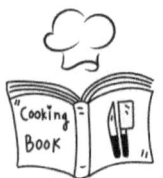

DIRECTIONS:

1

Combine dill, olive oil, lemon juice, honey, garlic, coriander, salt, and pepper in a small bowl.

2

Rinse salmon fillet under running cold water and pat dry with paper towels. Lay salmon skin-side down on a large piece of plastic wrap. Spread dill mixture all over the top of the fish, wrap well with plastic wrap, and refrigerate for 30 minutes.

3

Preheat the oven to 425 degrees F (220 degrees C). Unwrap salmon and place skin-side down in a baking dish.

4

Bake in the preheated oven until salmon flakes easily with a fork, 12 to 15 minutes.

NUTRITION FACTS:

284 calories; protein 35.1g; carbohydrates 5.7g; fat 13.3g;

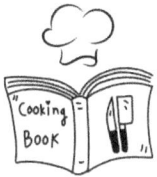

HERB-STUFFED BAKED TROUT

Prep:
15 mins
Cook:
20 mins
Total:
35 mins
Servings:
4
Yield:
4 servings

INGREDIENTS:

3 sprigs fresh parsley, or to taste
4 leaves fresh sage, or to taste
3 sprigs fresh dill, or to taste
1 lemon, thinly sliced
1 whole trout - cleaned, rinsed, and patted dry
2 tablespoons olive oil
salt and freshly ground black pepper to taste

DIRECTIONS:

1

Preheat the oven to 400 degrees F (200 degrees C).

2

Rub trout with olive oil, salt, and pepper. Rub the cavity of the trout with salt and stuff with parsley, sage, and dill. Make a few slits in the skin on the back of the trout and stuff with lemon slices. Place trout on a lined baking sheet.

3

Bake in preheated oven until flesh flakes easily with a fork, 20 to 30 minutes. Cover with aluminum foil if top starts browning too quickly.

NUTRITION FACTS:

200 calories; protein 18.7g; carbohydrates 4.4g; fat 12.7g; cholesterol 49.2mg; sodium 96.2mg

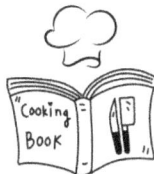

SHRIMP TERIYAKI

Prep:
10 mins
Cook:
20 mins
Total:
30 mins
Servings:
6
Yield:
6 servings

INGREDIENTS:

⅓ cup brown sugar
1 teaspoon sesame seeds
½ cup white wine
3 tablespoons teriyaki sauce, or more to taste
½ cup teriyaki marinade
2 (16 ounce) packages frozen deluxe stir-fry vegetables
2 cups hot cooked white rice
2 tablespoons olive oil
40 uncooked medium shrimp
2 cloves crushed garlic
⅛ teaspoon garlic powder
⅛ teaspoon ground ginger

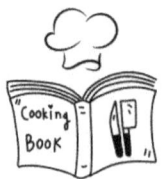

DIRECTIONS:

1

Heat oil in a wok over medium heat. Add shrimp, garlic, garlic powder, and ginger. Cook until shrimp are opaque, 3 to 5 minutes.

2

Add brown sugar and sesame seeds. Blend in white wine, teriyaki sauce, and teriyaki marinade and bring to a boil. Add frozen vegetables and return to a boil. Reduce heat to a simmer. Cover and cook until vegetables are heated through and tender, 10 to 15 minutes.

3

Serve stir-fry over a bed of rice.

NUTRITION FACTS:

354 calories; protein 19.5g; carbohydrates 53.4g; fat 6.3g; cholesterol 101.4mg;

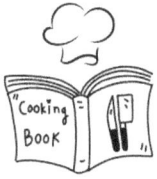

CHAPTER 5: SALAD RECIPES

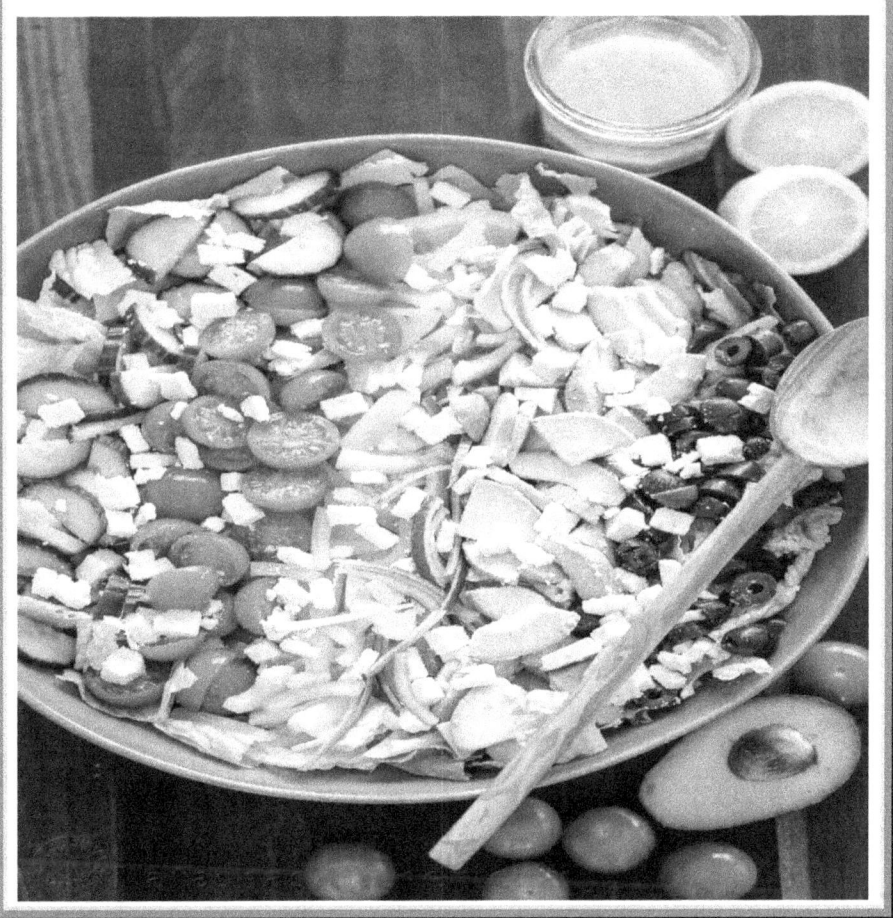

BOW-TIE PASTA SALAD

Prep:
20 mins
Cook:
15 mins
Additional:
3 hrs
Total:
3 hrs 35 mins
Servings:
12
Yield:
12 servings

INGREDIENTS:

1 (16 ounce) package bow-tie pasta (farfalle)
1 (12 ounce) bag broccoli florets
1 (10 ounce) basket cherry or grape tomatoes
1 bunch green onions, sliced
½ cup chopped celery
½ red bell pepper, chopped
½ green bell pepper, chopped
2 cups creamy salad dressing (such as Miracle Whip®)
⅓ cup grated Parmesan cheese
¼ cup white sugar
½ teaspoon dried basil
½ teaspoon salt

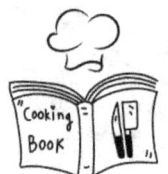

DIRECTIONS:

1

Bring a large pot of lightly salted water to a rolling boil. Cook the bow-tie pasta at a boil until tender yet firm to the bite, about 12 minutes; drain.

2

Quickly rinse the cooked pasta in cold water to stop it from continuing to cook; drain.

3

Mix the cooled pasta, broccoli, tomatoes, sliced green onions, celery, red bell pepper, and green bell pepper in a large bowl.

4

Gently stir the salad dressing, Parmesan cheese, sugar, basil, and salt in a bowl until evenly mixed.

5

Pour the salad dressing mixture over the pasta mixture; gently toss to coat evenly.

6

Refrigerate 3 hours to overnight before serving

NUTRITION FACTS:

317 calories; protein 7.7g; carbohydrates 43.5g; fat 12.4g;

BLACK BEAN AND WILD RICE SALAD

Prep:
20 mins
Additional:
30 mins
Total:
50 mins
Servings:
8
Yield:
8 servings

INGREDIENTS:

½ cup freshly squeezed orange juice
¼ cup olive oil
3 tablespoons tarragon vinegar
1 ½ teaspoons Dijon mustard
½ teaspoon dried thyme
¼ teaspoon ground cumin
⅛ teaspoon cayenne pepper
salt and ground black pepper to taste
1 red onion, finely chopped
1 bunch cilantro, chopped
1 (14 ounce) can black beans, drained and rinsed
1 (16 ounce) package cooked wild rice

½ cup dried cranberries

½ cup roughly chopped cashews

DIRECTIONS:

1

Toss the red onion, cilantro, black beans, wild rice, dried cranberries, and cashews together in a large mixing bowl.

2

Whisk the orange juice, olive oil, tarragon vinegar, Dijon mustard, thyme, cumin, cayenne pepper, salt, and black pepper together in a small bowl; pour over the rice mixture in the mixing bowl and toss to coat. Chill 30 minutes.

NUTRITION FACTS:

253 calories; protein 7g; carbohydrates 32.8g; fat 11.4g;

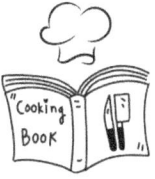

RICED CAULIFLOWER

Prep:
10 mins
Cook:
10 mins
Total:
20 mins
Servings:
2
Yield:
2 servings

INGREDIENTS:

salt and ground black pepper to taste
1 cup salsa
2 green onions, sliced
2 tablespoons olive oil
1 head cauliflower, grated

DIRECTIONS:

1

Heat olive oil in a large skillet over medium heat. Add cauliflower and cook until tender, about 10 minutes; season with salt and pepper. Stir salsa and green onions into cauliflower.

NUTRITION FACTS:

231 calories; protein 8g; carbohydrates 24.4g; fat 14g;

PERSIMMON AND POMEGRANATE SALAD

Prep:
15 mins
Cook:
10 mins
Additional:
30 mins
Total:
55 mins
Servings:
4

INGREDIENTS:

½ cup pecan halves
½ lime, juiced
7 fresh tarragon leaves, thinly sliced crosswise, or more to taste
salt and ground black pepper to taste
1 (8 ounce) package herb salad mix
2 Fuyu persimmons, peeled and each cut into 8 pieces
1 large pomegranate, peeled and seeds separated
¾ cup orange juice, divided
2 teaspoons cornstarch
1 ½ tablespoons honey
¼ cup extra-virgin olive oil

DIRECTIONS:

1

Preheat oven to 375 degrees F (190 degrees C).

2

Spread pecans onto a baking sheet.

3

Bake pecans in the preheated oven until toasted and fragrant, 5 to 7 minutes. Set aside to cool.

4

Whisk 1/2 cup orange juice and cornstarch together in a small saucepan; cook and stir over medium heat until mixture thickens, 3 to 5 minutes. Remove saucepan from heat and stir in honey until dissolved. Stir remaining 1/4 cup orange juice, olive oil, lime juice, tarragon leaves, salt, and pepper into orange juice mixture. Chill dressing in refrigerator, at least 30 minutes.

5

Spread herb salad mix into a serving bowl or on individual plates; top with persimmon slices, pomegranate seeds, and pecans. Drizzle cooled dressing over salad.

NUTRITION FACTS:

354 calories; protein 3.5g; carbohydrates 33.1g; fat 25.2g; sodium 56.4mg

MEXICAN MANGO SALAD

Prep:
35 mins
Total:
35 mins
Servings:
4

INGREDIENTS:

2 avocados, cut into cubes
20 cherry tomatoes, halved
1 mango, cubed
2 cups mixed salad greens
2 cups bite-size pieces of romaine lettuce
½ red onion, chopped
3 green onions, chopped

Dressing:

4 limes, juiced
2 tablespoons olive oil
1 tablespoon white sugar
¼ teaspoon ground red pepper
¼ teaspoon ground cumin
¼ teaspoon salt
¼ teaspoon ground black pepper

DIRECTIONS:

1

Combine avocados, tomatoes, mango, mixed greens, romaine lettuce, red onion, and green onions in a bowl. Toss salad until evenly mixed.

2

Combine lime juice, olive oil, sugar, red pepper, cumin, salt, and black pepper in a separate bowl. Whisk dressing until blended. Pour into the salad; toss briefly and serve.

NUTRITION FACTS:

314 calories; protein 4.5g; carbohydrates 33.1g; fat 22.2g;

PEAR SALAD

Prep:
15 mins
Cook:
10 mins
Additional:
1 hr
Total:
1 hr 25 mins
Servings:
12
Yield:
12 servings

INGREDIENTS:

1 (29 ounce) can pears in juice, juice drained and reserved
1 (3 ounce) package lemon-flavored gelatin mix
1 (8 ounce) package cream cheese, softened
2 tablespoons milk
1 (12 ounce) container frozen whipped topping thawed

DIRECTIONS:

1

Mash pears with a fork in a bowl until desired consistency is reached.

2

Measure 1 1/2 cups juice from pears and pour into a saucepan; cook over medium-low heat until warmed, 5 to 10 minutes. Remove saucepan from heat and stir gelatin mix into pear juice until dissolved. Stir cream cheese and milk into gelatin mixture until smooth. Fold whipped topping into mixture; add pears and mix well. Spoon mixture into a 9x9-inch baking dish. Refrigerate until set, at least 1 hour.

CHAPTER 6:
MEAT
RECIPES

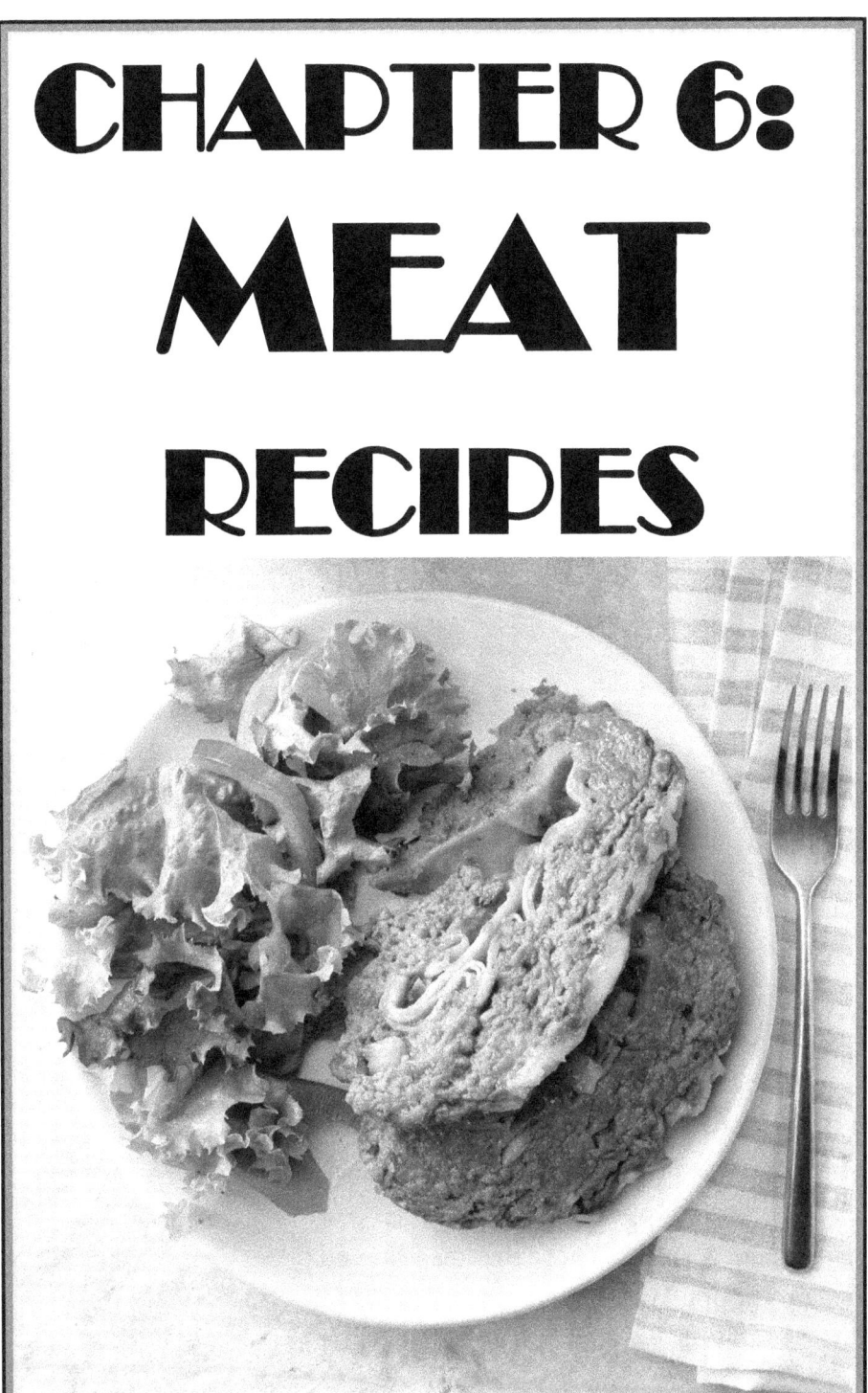

RICE SALAD

Prep:
20 mins
Cook:
30 mins
Additional:
4 hrs
Total:
4 hrs 50 mins
Servings:
8
Yield:
8 servings

INGREDIENTS:

2 cups water
1 cup white rice
6 eggs
1 tablespoon lemon juice
¼ cup sweet pickle relish
1 (9 ounce) can solid white tuna packed in water, drained
¼ teaspoon dried dill weed
1 teaspoon salt
⅛ teaspoon pepper
1 (10 ounce) package frozen peas, thawed
1 cup chopped celery
¼ cup chopped onion

1 (4 ounce) jar diced pimento

1 cup mayonnaise

1 teaspoon prepared mustard

DIRECTIONS:

1

In a saucepan bring water to a boil. Add rice and stir. Reduce heat, cover and simmer for 20 minutes. Remove from heat, and set aside to cool.

2

Place eggs in a saucepan and cover with cold water. Bring to a boil and immediately remove from heat. Cover and let eggs stand in hot water for 10 to 12 minutes. Remove from hot water, cool, peel and chop.

3

Rinse frozen peas under cold water. Strain, and place in a large mixing bowl. Add eggs, rice, celery, onions, and pimiento; toss to combine, and set aside. In a separate bowl, stir the mayonnaise together with mustard, lemon juice, relish, tuna, dill, salt, and pepper until well blended. Add to the vegetable mixture, and toss to combine. Cover, and refrigerate for a minimum of 4 hours. Toss once more before serving. Serve chilled.

NUTRITION FACTS:

424 calories; protein 17.2g; carbohydrates 30.1g; fat 26.2g; cholesterol 158.8mg

ORZO AND WILD RICE SALAD

Prep:
15 mins
Cook:
25 mins
Additional:
2 hrs 20 mins
Total:
3 hrs
Servings:
4
Yield:
4 servings

INGREDIENTS:

½ cup wild rice
2 cups water
1 cup orzo pasta
3 tablespoons chopped red onion
3 tablespoons dried currants
2 tablespoons chopped fresh basil
½ teaspoon salt
½ teaspoon ground black pepper
2 tablespoons white balsamic vinegar
1 ½ tablespoons honey

¾ teaspoon Dijon mustard
¼ teaspoon minced garlic
⅛ teaspoon pepper
1 ½ teaspoons chopped fresh basil
¼ cup canola oil
¼ cup extra-virgin olive oil
2 tablespoons corn kernels, drained
3 tablespoons diced yellow bell pepper
3 tablespoons diced red bell pepper
3 tablespoons diced green bell pepper

DIRECTIONS:

1

Bring the wild rice and water to a boil in a saucepan. Reduce heat to medium-low, cover, and simmer until the rice is tender but not mushy, 20 to 45 minutes depending on the variety of wild rice. Drain off any excess liquid, fluff the rice with a fork, and cook uncovered 5 minutes more. Once finished, spread into a shallow dish, and refrigerate until cold.

2

Bring a large pot of lightly salted water to a boil. Add the orzo pasta, and cook until al dente, 7 to 8 minute. Drain, rinse with cold water, and chill.

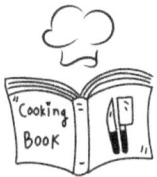

3

Place the chilled rice and orzo into a large mixing bowl. Stir in the red onion, currants, corn, yellow bell pepper, red bell pepper, and green bell pepper. Season with 2 tablespoons basil, salt, and 1/2 teaspoon pepper. In a separate bowl, whisk together the vinegar, honey, mustard, garlic, 1/8 teaspoon pepper, and 1 1/2 teaspoons basil. Slowly whisk in the canola and olive oils until emulsified. Stir the dressing into the pasta, and refrigerate 2 hours before serving.

NUTRITION FACTS:

566 calories; protein 10.6g; carbohydrates 68.2g; fat 29.1g;

COUSCOUS WITH A KICK

Prep:
20 mins
Cook:
10 mins
Total:
30 mins
Servings:
6
Yield:
6 servings

INGREDIENTS:

1 clove garlic, minced
½ cup chopped green onion
3 tablespoons chopped fresh mint
3 tablespoons chopped fresh basil
3 tablespoons chopped fresh cilantro
1 tablespoon chopped fresh parsley
2 teaspoons ground cumin
2 teaspoons cayenne pepper
1 lemon, juiced
3 cups water
2 cups couscous
½ cup crumbled feta cheese
1 fresh jalapeno pepper, chopped
½ cucumber, diced

DIRECTIONS:

1

Bring the water to a boil in a saucepan. Remove from the heat and stir in the couscous. Cover and let stand until the couscous absorbs the water entirely, about 10 minutes; fluff with a fork.

2

While the couscous soaks, stir the feta cheese, jalapeno pepper, cucumber, garlic, green onion, mint, basil, cilantro, parsley, cumin, cayenne pepper, and lemon juice in a large bowl. Add the prepared couscous and mix well.

NUTRITION FACTS:

210 calories; protein 8.1g; carbohydrates 38.3g; fat 3.3g; cholesterol 11.1mg; sodium 155mg.

SMOTHERED PORK CHOPS

Servings:
6
Yield:
6 servings

INGREDIENTS:

6 (3/4 inch) thick pork chops
½ cup water
⅓ cup all-purpose flour
1 (14.5 ounce) can fat-free chicken broth
1 tablespoon browning sauce
1 onion, chopped
4 cloves crushed garlic

DIRECTIONS:

1
Saute onion and garlic in a non-stick skillet coated with vegetable spray until tender. Add pork chops, and brown on both sides. Add 1/2 cup of water, and bring to a boil.

2
Whisk together, flour, chicken broth, and browning sauce until smooth. Add to skillet, stirring well. Cover and cook over low heat 30 to 45 minutes or until tender.

NUTRITION FACTS:

187 calories; protein 25.8g; carbohydrates 7.8g; fat 5.2g;

CHEESY PORK CHOPS WITH SPICY APPLES

Prep:
15 mins
Cook:
20 mins
Total:
35 mins
Servings:
4
Yield:
4 servings

INGREDIENTS:

2 teaspoons white sugar
2 tablespoons balsamic vinegar
4 pork chops
salt and pepper to taste
4 slices extra sharp Cheddar cheese
1 tablespoon butter
1 onion, sliced
1 pinch red pepper flakes
1 apple, cored and sliced

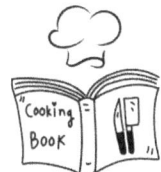

DIRECTIONS:

1

Prepare a grill for high heat.

2

While the grill heats, melt the butter in a skillet over medium heat. Add the onion, and cook until soft. Season with red pepper flakes then add the sliced apple. Stir in the sugar and balsamic vinegar, and simmer for 5 minutes, or until apples are soft and golden.

3

Season the pork chops with salt and pepper. Grill for 3 to 5 minutes per side, depending on thickness. Spoon the onions and apples on top of the chops, and top with a slice of Cheddar cheese. Cover the grill, and cook for about 3 minutes until cheese is melted and bubbling.

NUTRITION FACTS:

301 calories; protein 22.1g; carbohydrates 11.7g; fat 18.7g;

GROUND BEEF AND CHOPPED CABBAGE

Prep:
10 mins
Cook:
35 mins
Total:
45 mins
Servings:
10
Yield:
10 servings

INGREDIENTS:

1 tablespoon olive oil
1 large onion, chopped
1 ½ pounds ground beef
1 teaspoon garlic powder
½ teaspoon red pepper flakes
½ teaspoon Italian seasoning
salt and pepper to taste
1 small head cabbage, chopped
2 (14.5 ounce) cans diced tomatoes
1 (14.5 ounce) can tomato sauce

DIRECTIONS:

1

Heat olive oil in a large heavy pot or a 6-quart Dutch oven over medium heat. Cook and stir onion in hot oil until translucent, about 5 minutes.

2

Break ground beef into small chunks and add to the pot; cook and stir, continuing to break the beef into smaller pieces, until the beef is completely browned, 5 to 7 minutes.

3

Season beef mixture with garlic powder, red pepper flakes, Italian seasoning, and a dash of salt. Stir cabbage, diced tomatoes, and tomato sauce with the beef mixture; bring to a boil, reduce heat to low, and cook mixture at a simmer until cabbage is fork-tender, about 25 minutes. Season with salt and pepper.

NUTRITION FACTS:

178 calories; protein 13.3g; carbohydrates 8.7g; fat 9.7g; cholesterol 42.6mg

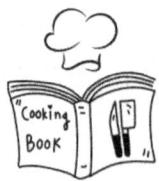

CHAPTER 7: SOUP & STEW RECIPES

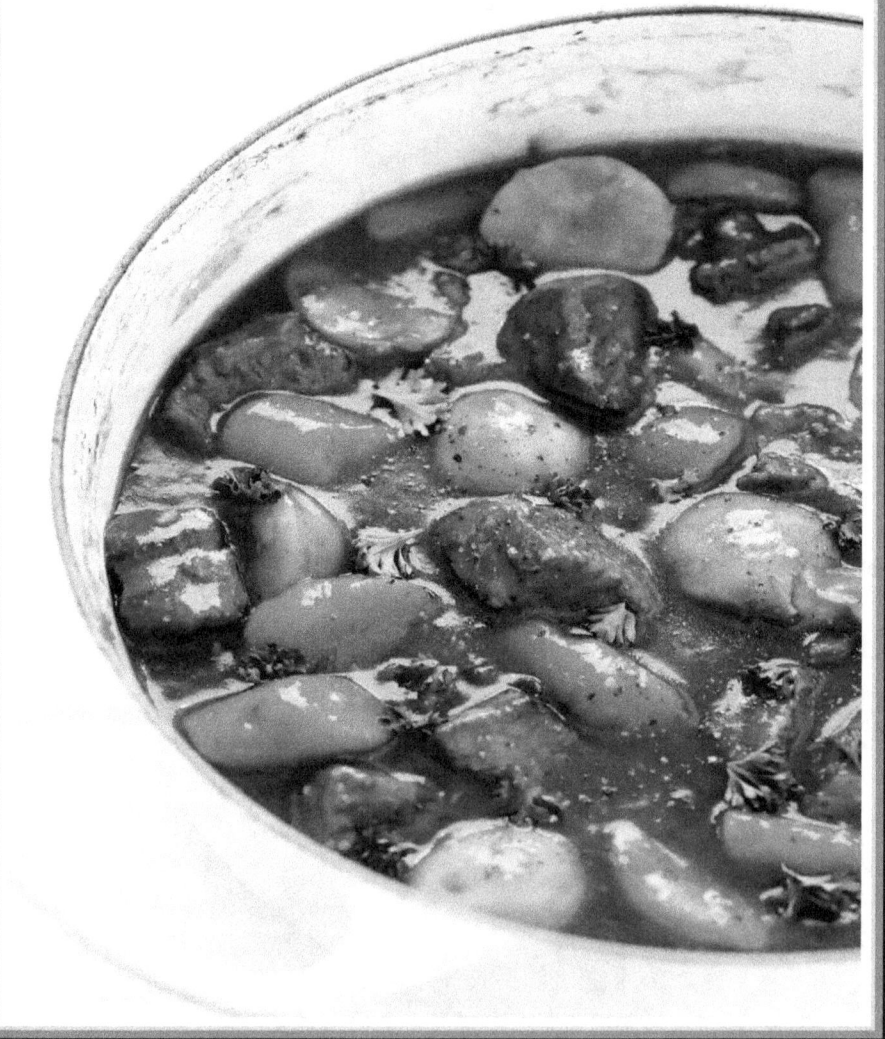

ROTISSERIE CHICKEN NOODLE SOUP

Prep:
25 mins
Cook:
25 mins
Total:
50 mins
Servings:
6
Yield:
6 servings

INGREDIENTS:

1 tablespoon olive oil
1 pound carrots, sliced diagonally
1 cup chopped celery
½ medium yellow onion, chopped
1 teaspoon dried oregano
1 teaspoon Italian seasoning
½ teaspoon seasoned salt
salt and ground black pepper to taste
2 cloves garlic, minced
4 cups chicken broth, or to taste
1 (8 ounce) package extra-wide egg noodles
1 cooked rotisserie chicken - skinned, boned, and meat shredded

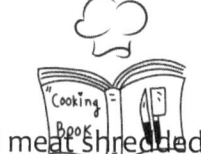

DIRECTIONS:

1

Coat the bottom of a Dutch oven with olive oil. Add carrots, celery, onion, oregano, Italian seasoning, seasoned salt, salt, and pepper. Saute over medium-high heat until vegetables have softened, 6 to 8 minutes. Add garlic and cook until onion is translucent and garlic scent has lessened slightly, about 4 to 5 minutes.

2

Add chicken broth and bring to a boil. Add egg noodles; cook 5 to 6 minutes. Gently stir in shredded chicken and simmer until egg noodles are tender and chicken is heated through, 2 to 3 more minutes. Serve immediately.

NUTRITION FACTS:

360 calories; protein 28.5g; carbohydrates 36.9g; fat 10.3g;

CHICKEN UDON NOODLE SOUP

Prep:
20 mins
Cook:
15 mins
Total:
35 mins
Servings:
4
Yield:
4 servings

INGREDIENTS:

1 large cooked skinless, boneless chicken breast, chopped
1 head bok choy, chopped
¼ cup dried shiitake mushrooms
2 (7 ounce) packages dried udon noodles
½ cup mung bean sprouts
1 green onion, sliced diagonally
2 tablespoons dried minced onion
1 tablespoon chopped fresh cilantro
1 ½ (32 fluid ounce) containers chicken stock
1 clove garlic, minced
1 tablespoon minced fresh ginger root
1 teaspoon chili powder

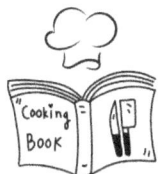

DIRECTIONS:

1

Bring chicken stock, garlic, ginger, and chili powder to a boil in a pot over medium-high heat. Add chicken, bok choy, and mushrooms; let simmer lightly for 3 minutes. Add noodles and cook soup for 4 minutes more.

2

Pour soup mixture evenly into 2 soup bowls. Place mung beans on top in the center of each bowl, with green onion placed neatly on top. Sprinkle dried onions and cilantro on top.

NUTRITION FACTS:

507 calories; protein 23.7g; carbohydrates 88.1g; fat 6.7g;

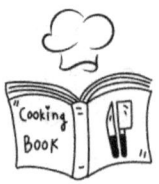

AMAZING OVEN-BRAISED CHICKEN STEW

Prep:
30 mins
Cook:
55 mins
Total:
1 hr 25 mins
Servings:
8
Yield:
8 servings

INGREDIENTS:

1 (16 ounce) package fresh mushrooms, quartered
3 cups trimmed and chopped fresh green beans
2 tablespoons minced garlic
¾ cup dry white wine
3 cups chicken broth, or as needed
2 sprigs fresh rosemary, or to taste
3 tablespoons cornstarch
2 tablespoons water, or as needed
2 pounds boneless, skinless chicken thighs
salt and ground black pepper to taste
1 tablespoon extra-virgin olive oil
1 tablespoon unsalted butter

2 cups chopped onions
3 cups chopped carrots
1 ½ cups chopped celery

DIRECTIONS:

1

Preheat the oven to 350 degrees F (175 degrees C).

2

Cut each chicken thigh into 5 or 6 pieces. Lightly season with salt and pepper.

3

Heat oil and butter in a 6-quart, oven-safe Dutch oven over medium-high heat until hot. Add chicken pieces and cook until lightly browned but not cooked through, about 2 minutes per side. Remove chicken from the pot with a slotted spoon and set aside.

4

Add onions to the hot pot; cook and stir for 1 minute. Add carrots and celery; cook, stirring occasionally, for 1 more minute. Add mushrooms and cook for 1 minute. Add green beans and garlic; cook and stir until fragrant, about 2 minutes. Season lightly with salt and pepper to taste.

5
Pour wine into the pot and bring to a boil while scraping the browned bits of food off the bottom of the pan with a wooden spoon. Add chicken and any accumulated juices back to the pot. Pour in just enough chicken broth to barely cover everything in the pot. Sample broth and adjust seasonings, if necessary. Add rosemary sprigs, pressing them below the surface of the liquid.

6
Cover and place in the center of the preheated oven. Bake until vegetables are tender and chicken is no longer pink in the center and the juices run clear, about 30 minutes. An instant-read thermometer inserted into the center should read at least 165 degrees F (74 degrees C). Remove rosemary sprigs.

7
Place cornstarch in a small bowl and add just enough water to create a thin paste. Stir until all lumps are dissolved and slowly add to the stew, stirring constantly.

8
Place stew on the stove and heat over medium heat. Cook and stir until gravy has thickened and desired consistency has been achieved, about 5 minutes.

NUTRITION FACTS:

310 calories; protein 21.9g; carbohydrates 18.3g; fat 15g;

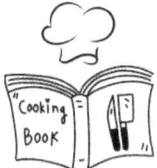

HEALTHY ROASTED CAULIFLOWER SOUP

Prep:
10 mins
Cook:
30 mins
Total:
40 mins
Servings:
4

INGREDIENTS:

1 large head cauliflower, broken into florets
2 medium white onions, cut in half lengthwise and thinly sliced
3 tablespoons olive oil
1 ½ teaspoons ground cumin
1 ½ teaspoons ground coriander
1 teaspoon salt
½ teaspoon ground black pepper
2 tablespoons salted butter
4 cloves garlic, crushed
1 large potato, with skin, cut into 1-inch pieces
1 teaspoon ground turmeric
1 quart vegetable stock
2 tablespoons sliced almonds

DIRECTIONS:

1

Preheat the oven to 400 degrees F (200 degrees C).

2

Spread out cauliflower and onion on a baking sheet. Drizzle with olive oil and season with cumin, coriander, salt and pepper. Toss to combine.

3

Roast vegetables in the preheated oven until cauliflower is browned and cooked, but not soft, about 25 minutes.

4

Meanwhile, melt butter in a large saucepan over low heat. Add garlic and cook until fragrant, about 3 minutes. Stir in potato and turmeric. Pour in stock, increase heat to medium, and bring to a simmer. Cover and cook until potato is soft, about 10 minutes.

5

Set aside 1 cup roasted cauliflower for topping. Add remaining cauliflower and onion to the soup and return to a simmer. Cook for 5 minutes for flavors to meld. Puree with an immersion blender or food processor until soup is smooth. Adjust seasoning to taste.

6

Toast the almonds in a dry skillet over low heat, stirring occasionally, until golden.

7
Ladle soup into bowls, and top with reserved cauliflower and toasted almonds

NUTRITION FACTS:

329 calories; protein 8.2g; carbohydrates 36.4g; fat 18.7g;

www.ingramcontent.com/pod-product-compliance
Lightning Source LLC
Chambersburg PA
CBHW070931080526
44589CB00013B/1470